I0439396

Sugar-Free Smoothies For The Fast Diet

Alicia Brent

ISBN: 149736423X
ISBN-13: 978-1497364233

Also by Alicia Brent

Samuel Johnson – Man of Words

Scraps of Food

A Little Book of Christmas: An Abundance of Quotes
for the Festive Season

Resolutions and Reflections for the New Year

Ellen White Speaks Out

Chapters

Page

Introduction

I am beginning with the assumption that you are already somewhat familiar with the concept of the Fast Diet (sometimes called the 5:2 or Intermittent Fasting Diet), which basically involves cutting your calorie intake, on just two days each week, to a quarter of the normal daily allowance. So that means 500 calories for women and 600 for men.

I will shortly tell you about my experience of this increasingly popular, successful and extremely do-able diet (eighteen months and counting in my case), which is really not so much a diet as a completely new way of eating that actually does work.

We'll also have a look at the dangers, often hidden, lurking in the bitter-sweet sugar trap that many of us, quite unwittingly, get drawn into as we shop, under the illusion that we are buying healthy foods.

And finally, I'll describe how sugar-free smoothies became an important aspect of my approach to the fast days, making this regime even more simple, varied and enjoyable to follow.

But first a bit about myself...

I grew up in a close-knit, loving family in rural Yorkshire.

Yet my early school life was not a happy one as I quickly became a target for the school bullies on account of my size. Children can be extremely unkind to anyone who does not 'fit in'. As well as being on the podgy side I was also painfully shy and could never stand up for myself.

Instead of complaining to anyone I turned to food for comfort, particularly anything sweet. In fact, I took refuge in eating to such an extent that by the time I was a teenager I was terribly overweight and very self conscious about it. But rather than address my weight issues I ate even more, often in secret.

Academically though, I did well and with plenty of encouragement from my parents I passed every exam with flying colours, eventually securing a place at university. The name-calling and other forms of taunting had stopped by this time but, despite my success, my self esteem had reached rock bottom.

Although I had friends, I was socially anxious and preferred to spend much of my free time studying when they were out having fun. Nevertheless, I did begin to diet. I tried out lots of different diets and I did lose weight. However, the problem was that I could never stick to a particular diet for long, a few months being my limit on any one of the many I embarked on. I would give up for several months before attempting another weight loss regime. And so began my seemingly endless cycle of yo-yo dieting.

Fast forwarding twelve years found me married to Andrew, one of the kindest men on this planet and with two beautiful young children. I am five feet four inches tall but two years ago I weighed in at an unhealthy sixteen and a half stone (231 pounds) with a body mass index quite obviously well above the twenty-five level that's normal for a thirty year old woman. It didn't help that I did little to shed the thirty or so extra pounds I had piled on after my pregnancies.

Andrew has never been critical of my size but that didn't stop me feeling bad about myself. And since he was also somewhat overweight a couple of years back we both determined to lose weight together. The challenge was how to make a long-term commitment to a diet that we could sustain without too much difficulty. Fortunately for us, at this crucially decisive moment we became aware of the Fast Diet, which sounded immensely impressive. Having looked at all the available evidence about the numerous possible health benefits such as protection against Alzheimer's, Parkinson's disease and cancer, lowering cholesterol, regulating blood sugar, avoiding diabetes and the potential to live a much longer, active, healthy life, quite apart from the anticipated weight loss, we were convinced that this was indeed our best option.

Experiencing the Fast Diet

We began following the principles of the Fast Diet enthusiastically, trying out different ways before finding one that suited our lifestyles.

Initially, on our two fast days we ate nothing during the daytime but drank lots of calorie-free green tea and water, saving up all our allotted allowance for a decent meal in the evening.   Since Andrew and I are both vegetarians it was not difficult to fill our plates with a good sized portion each. In fact, we often found that we ended up leaving food, which was not only wasteful but also not a particularly good example for the children. And if we ate everything anyway, we felt bloated and uncomfortable. So we decided to have a smallish breakfast each day, leaving roughly 300 calories for an early supper, which worked well.

After attempting the two fast days back-to-back during the week, we realised that spreading them out gave us more choice to juggle them around social events like meals out, when we didn't want to restrict the calories. We frequently ended up with Mondays and Thursday as diet days.

Before we began the diet I thought I would be tempted to eat more than usual on my non-diet days and I did – but only in the early days, because I soon discovered that I actually could not manage as much on the day after a fast day as I thought I could. My eyes were larger than my stomach! So I learned to listen more carefully to my body.

When we were still getting used to this new way of eating, tiredness was a bit of a problem; yet after just a month, we were surprised to find that our energy levels were considerably higher than before we started. Feeling more energized and with a marked weight loss, we felt motivated to use our gym membership regularly which meant that we then lost even more weight!

Another plus for me was the improvement in my skin. Spots on my face, which had plagued me since the teenage years, magically disappeared. And when friends and family complimented me on my glowing complexion in addition to my new slimmer look, I knew I was was on the right track to a much healthier and hopefully, longer life. Slowly my sense of self esteem improved; I felt much happier and definitely more confident.

Whenever I have lapsed slightly Andrew has been there to support me - and vice versa.

My weight has finally dropped to a healthy ten stone, one pound (141 pounds) and Andrew is very proud of himself, having lost three and a half stone (49 pounds).

We will soon have been following and enjoying the Fast Diet for two years - something I honestly never thought I could possibly achieve.

The Sugar Trap

Sugar can be highly addictive. It's certainly high in calories, with a hefty intake resulting in massive weight gain and terrible tooth decay.

I do not want to preach about sugar; I am speaking from my personal bitter experience of the effects of consuming too much sweet stuff when I was younger and realised little about its dangers. I just knew that if I felt down it comforted me so I became habituated to eating candies, biscuits, cakes...

I put up with my expanding waistline, poor skin and frequent trips to the dentist, preferring to indulge my passion for something that seemed to make me feel better.

Research has shown that sugar consumption triggers a greater release of serotonin and dopamine – both feel-good chemicals – in the brain. However, shortly afterwards the level of these 'happy hormones' drops to lower than it was previously. In the same way as a drug would, this has a kind of 'withdrawal' effect, which means we crave it even more in order to replenish the 'missing' hormones.

Interestingly, strenuous exercise has the same effect as sugar, producing a similar 'high'.

When we eat sugar it either ends up being burnt for energy, which is obviously a good thing; or it is converted to glucose and stored in fat cells – not such great news.

Everyone knows that eating anything to excess is not sensible. Added to the harm outlined above, a constant overload of sugar is implicated in a number of serious conditions such as diabetes or an impaired immune system, as well as increasing the risk of some cancers, heart disease and polycystic ovarian syndrome.

One of the biggest problems with sugar is that it can be extremely hard to work out what our intake is. Whilst we are well aware of how much table sugar we add to our food and drinks it's not always clear, unless we carefully check every label, just how much sugar manufacturers are putting in the products we put into our shopping trolley.

And we could be fooled by the fact that sugar comes in many guises – sucrose, lactose, dextrose, maltose...

The real problem is refined sugar, the type usually found in our homes. This has been factory-processed and contains nothing of any nutritional value - no vitamins, proteins or fibre - but is full of calories.   Hence the expression "empty calories".

We know that biscuits and cakes contain a high amount of sugar but what about the hidden sugar in food?   Sauces, salad dressings (especially low fat ones), flavoured yoghurts, breakfast cereals, canned vegetables and soups, so-called health bars like granola, bread, ready-meals, together with concentrated fruit juices are among the numerous alluring culprits lurking on our supermarket/food store shelves. Take a look at the ingredients in some of the foods in your kitchen – you may be amazed or even shocked by the quantity of sugar in a few of them.

So what can you use instead?

A large number of sugar substitutes including agave, aspartame, sorbitol, saccharin and erythritol, although providing fewer calories, often cause unpleasant symptoms like bloating, diarrhoea and flatulence.

Stevia, on the other hand, is extracted from the leaf of a naturally sweet South American herb and Lo han (or luohangu) is a natural sweetener which is derived from a Chinese fruit. The latter is not widely available whereas Stevia is readily found alongside the sugar in your grocery store.

Not all sugars are bad for us, however. Fruits contain a naturally-occurring form of sugar known as fructose, which researchers have found does not trigger a sudden fluctuation in blood sugar since it is digested at a slower rate than sucrose. Sweeter-tasting fruits like peaches and cherries generally contain a greater amount of natural sugar whereas tarter fruits such as lemons have less; but very few fruits contain sufficient sugar to do you any harm whatsoever.

And when you eat fruit you are also consuming lots of important fibre (essential for healthy bowel functioning) as well as water and loads of vital health-giving vitamins and minerals.

Whilst there is no added sugar in any of the smoothies presented here, you will nevertheless find plenty of sweetness, sometimes in the form of stevia but also in the form of honey. This is not "cheating" – honey has many beneficial properties as well as scoring well on the Glycemic Index. However, to get the best from honey it should be stressed that processed, refined honeys, like so many processed foods, lack the benefits that can be gained from using the raw form. This may take a little more seeking out but it's worth it. Alternatively, use Manuka honey – an expensive alternative but one with, among other things, natural antibiotic properties.

A few words about the Glycemic Index are appropriate here. It's a measure of how quickly sugars are absorbed into the bloodstream, measured against glucose, which is absorbed rapidly and can cause a "spike" or sugar rush when taken in large quantities. Glucose is set at a score of 100 and other foods are measured against it as a percentage. Anything below 55 on this index is considered low – in other words, its sugar is absorbed slowly, allowing the body to cope with it comfortably. Raw and Manuka honeys score particularly well on the Glycemic Index,.

Similarly, the natural sugars found in fruit score well on this index; and, of course, fruit and vegetables also contain between them an enormous range of nutrients and roughage, which keep the body in healthy balance. Note that word *balance*. Our bodies need a balance of nutrients, *including* sugars. The problem in recent years has been an *overbalance* in favour of *added* sugar.

Using cinnamon adds an extra layer of sweetness whilst adding little in the way of calories.

Dieting Smoothiely

Relaxing at a sunny poolside during a summer holiday in Italy, sipping contentedly on a delightful fruit smoothie, I wished, as many of us often do at such times, that I could freeze the moment for all eternity. Sadly, or maybe fortunately, time moved on regardless. But not before an inspiring thought hit me:

Why not use smoothies as a regular part of my diet?

I may not always be able to have the sun, or a sun bed by a swimming pool. But I could re-create the feeling of contentment by enjoying a smoothie whenever I wanted; and it would add a lot of exciting variety to my fast days.
Back home in England I started collecting ideas, making sure that all my smoothies used no added sugar and that pure fruit juices were kept to a sensible level (all things in moderation!). I experimented with interesting combinations, using vegetables as well as fruit, keeping a written record of anything that worked. Andrew, at first dubious that a low calorie smoothie would be satisfying enough

as a meal substitute, became equally enthusiastic and started trying out ideas of his own.

One great advantage of dieting the smoothie way was that the preparation of the meal was much quicker, and generally easier, than cooking. All we needed were a blender and a couple of tall glasses – plus, of course, the ingredients, which for the most part, were to be found in the freezer or refrigerator. Even the most complicated smoothie took only minutes to prepare.

We took it in turns to produce our smoothies and to make it more interesting we chose to surprise each other with whatever we made. On sunny days we sat outdoors on our patio – a particular pleasure at breakfast-time – to make the most of the experience.

All ingredients were, of course, calorie-counted and I carefully recorded the total for each smoothie on my record sheet.

Not only were the smoothies delicious (even the children love them), they were also very nutritious and satisfying and we now prefer them on our diet days to any other type of meal.

Having reached a total of fifty of these grand concoctions, I decided to incorporate them in a book and share my experiences with others. Whether dieting or not, I am quite sure that everyone will find much to enjoy in the recipes that follow.

You might well raise an eyebrow or two at first glance: some of the ingredients may seem strange bedfellows. Who in their right mind would think of mixing peas with strawberries? Well, me, for one! In fact, when my youngest son tasted that particular smoothie ("Fruity Pea") he asked for more; and he doesn't even like peas!

There has always been a blurring of the edges between sweet and savoury foods. Think of those cocktail sticks at parties, holding a mix of cheese, pickled onions and pineapple. And although carrot is usually regarded as a savoury food, carrot cake is widely enjoyed, as is a mixture of carrot and orange juice. Carrot is yet another sweetener as well as being a vegetable in its own right. So experimenting with apparently incompatible flavours is not such a crazy idea...

In order to make the most of your smoothies, a few notes of guidance follow:

If you don't already have a blender, choose carefully.

- Do you, for instance, want a glass or plastic container? Plastic is lighter but glass is more stable, scratch-proof and easier to clean.
- Make sure the pouring spout is wide and well rounded to make pouring easy and dripping less likely.
- Choose one with a more than a single speed (two are usually sufficient) and an ice-crushing capability.
- A pulse control is essential to dislodge any blockages.
- And make sure the motor is up to the job (400 watts or more).
- But don't pay more than you need by being tempted by facilities you don't need: there are even *sixteen* speed models available!
- Spend some time getting to know your blender's capabilities to get the best

from it.

- Depending on how well your blender copes with frozen or dense ingredients, you may wish to add them in small amounts, blending each addition before adding more. In the case of my aging blender I've found using the pulse control in brief bursts before using the speed settings particularly helpful in getting the results I want. Also, using the slow speed before increasing to the highest setting is generally more successful than going straight to high power.

Selecting and preparing ingredients:

- The riper the fruit, the easier it will be for the blender to process. Chop firm or hard ingredients (particularly carrot, celery and rhubarb) into small pieces to enable the blades to break them up more easily.

- Frozen fruit, if available, can be substituted for fresh (and vice versa). I often use frozen because it avoids a lot of mess (especially when using mango!), saves time and makes it easier to weigh out exactly the amounts I want. Calorie-wise there is no difference.

Putting you in control:

- Choosing the type of liquid content is up to you. You may be quite happy to follow the recipes as stated. But you may prefer to use water instead of milk (in which case deduct 3 calories per fluid ounce from your calorie total if the milk used is almond milk, or 11 calories per fl.oz if it's skimmed milk. You may also wish to switch between skimmed milk and almond milk. If you do, add 5 calories per fl.oz if using skimmed instead of almond, or subtract 5 if using almond over skimmed.

Thinning down:
- If you prefer a thinner consistency than a recipe makes, you can add a small amount of water, which is unlikely to affect the flavour significantly. Alternatively, if you have a few spare calories available for your smoothie,

you may wish to add a little almond milk (only 3 calories per fluid ounce (30ml).

Thickening:

- In a few cases I've used banana as a thickener as well as for its flavour. However, banana is quite high in calories (105 for a medium size and 70 for a small one). You can, if you prefer, either halve the banana amount to give a thinner consistency whilst still retaining banana flavouring, or leave out the banana altogether and use half a teaspoon of xanthan gum, which is a thickening agent but with only 10 calories per teaspoonful. Once again this enables you to control your calorie intake to suit yourself. Of course, this will not work where banana is the principal ingredient (the smoothie called "Simply Banana" would then become "Simply" – not a great name and not much flavour either!).

The recipes are set out in order of calorie content for ease of reference. I've also classified them at the end of the book into fruity, vegetable, and fruit and vegetable mixed.

You will notice that some of the recipes are for two servings, whilst others are for one. If you are following the Fast Diet with someone else, the two-serving amounts are ideal. If you make these for one person you can either store the second half in a sealed container overnight (refrigerated of course) or simply halve the quantities. If you do save your smoothie until the following day, do give it a good stir before drinking.

So now, all that remains is for me to wish you a "Happy Smoothieday."

Smoothie Recipes

Cocomelon

Ingredients:

240ml (8 fl.oz) coconut water

336g (12 oz) deseeded watermelon

Juice of ½ lime

3 mint leaves

Ice Cubes

Preparation:

- Pour coconut water into blender
- Add watermelon & lime juice
- Put in mint leaves
- Blend until smooth

Makes **two** servings

Calories per serving: 75

Blueberry Sparkle

Ingredients:

336g (12 oz) watermelon chunks, deseeded

150ml (5fl.oz) sparkling water

84g (3 oz) frozen blueberries

1 tablespoon fresh lime juice

4 mint leaves

Preparation:

- Put watermelon chunks into blender
- Add water
- Drop in blueberries & lime juice
- Throw in mint leaves
- Blend until smooth

Makes **two** servings

Calories per serving: 77

Fruity Watercress

Ingredients:

180ml (6 fl.oz) water

14g (½ oz) watercress

½ small banana

42g (1½ oz) blueberries

42g (1½ oz) chilled pineapple

Ice Cubes

Preparation:

- Pour water into blender
- Add watercress
- Slice & add banana
- Put in blueberries
- Cut pineapple into chunks &add
- Add ice cubes
- Blend to combine thoroughly

Makes **one** serving

Calories per serving: 79

Strawberry & Cucumber Cooler

Ingredients:

240ml (8fl.oz) unsweetened almond milk

½ cucumber

224g (8 oz) strawberries

1tablespoon honey

1 teaspoon pure lemon juice

Preparation:

- Pour almond milk into blender
- Peel cucumber, cut into chunks & add to blender
- Pop in strawberries
- Add honey & lemon juice
- Blend to a smooth consistency

Makes **two** servings

Calories per serving: 84

Rhubarb Rocker

Ingredients:

120ml (4 fl.oz) water

112g (4 oz) fat-free natural yoghurt

2 ripe sticks of ripe rhubarb

1 tablespoon pure orange juice

Stevia to taste

Ice cubes

Preparation:

- Pour water into blender
- Add yoghurt
- Chop & add rhubarb
- Pour in orange juice
- Add stevia & ice cubes
- Blend vigorously

Makes **one** serving

Calories per serving: 94

Celery & Blueberry

Ingredients:

180ml (6 fl.oz) unsweetened soya milk

84g (3 oz) blueberries

¼ teaspoon vanilla extract

1 stick celery

Stevia to taste

Ice cubes

Preparation:

- Pour soya milk into blender
- Add blueberries & vanilla extract
- Chop celery finely & add
- Pop in ice cubes & stevia
- Blend until everything is completely combined

Makes **one** serving

Calories per serving: 98

Passionate Minty Melon

Ingredients:

240ml (8 fl.oz) pure passion fruit juice

½ cucumber

168g (6 oz) honeydew melon

1 tablespoon chopped mint

Preparation:

- Pour passion fruit juice into blender
- Peel cucumber, cut into chunks & put into blender
- Add melon & mint
- Blend thoroughly

Makes **two** servings

Calories per serving: 100

Caribbean Calypso

Ingredients:

120ml (4 fl.oz) pure orange juice

120ml (4 fl.oz) pure pineapple juice

½ teaspoon fresh grated ginger root

½ teaspoon xanthan gum

Ice cubes

Preparation:

- Pour orange & pineapple juices into blender
- Add ginger root & xanthan gum
- Put in ice cubes
- Blend until everything is combined

Makes **one** serving

Calories per serving: 100

Strawberry Delight

Ingredients:

240ml (8 fl.oz) unsweetened almond milk

56g (2 oz) cottage cheese

84g (3 oz) frozen strawberries

Pinch cinnamon

Tiny pinch salt

Stevia to taste

Preparation:

- Pour almond milk into blender
- Add cottage cheese
- Blend briefly to aerate
- Add strawberries, cinnamon, salt & stevia
- Blend until smooth

Makes **one** serving

Calories per serving: 111

Purple Sunset

Ingredients:

120ml (4 fl.oz) pure cranberry juice

½ cucumber

84g (3 oz) blueberries

10g ($^1/_3$ oz) chopped parsley

Stevia to taste

Ice cubes

Preparation:

- Pour cranberry juice into blender
- Peel, chop & add cucumber
- Add blueberries & parsley
- Put in stevia to taste
- Drop in ice cubes
- Blend until all ingredients are completely combined

Makes **one** serving

Calories per serving: 112

Berry Mix

Ingredients:

240ml (8 fl.oz) unsweetened almond milk

168g (6 oz) blackberries

168g (6 oz) blueberries

168g (6 oz)) strawberries

Pinch ground cinnamon

Ice cubes

Preparation:

- Pour almond milk into blender
- Put in blackberries, blueberries & strawberries
- Add cinnamon & ice cubes
- Blend all ingredients thoroughly

Makes **two** servings

Calories per serving: 117

Pear & Strawberry

Ingredients:

180ml (6 fl.oz) unsweetened almond milk

1 ripe Asian pear

56g (2 oz) strawberries

56g (2 oz) fat-free natural yoghurt

Preparation:

- Pour milk into blender
- Chop & add pear
- Add strawberries
- Pour on yoghurt
- Blend until everything is combined

Makes **one** serving

Calories per serving: 118

Berry Nice

Ingredients:

120ml (4 fl.oz) unsweetened almond milk

140g (5 oz) frozen mixed berries

56g (2 oz) fat-free natural yoghurt

¼ teaspoon vanilla extract

Stevia to taste

Preparation:

- Pour milk into blender
- Put in berries
- Add yoghurt & vanilla extract
- Blend until everything is combined

Makes **one** serving

Calories per serving: 120

Pinkalicious

Ingredients:

240ml (8 fl.oz) unsweetened almond milk

1 teaspoon ground flax seed

112g (4 oz) raspberries

56g (2 oz) frozen cherries

Stevia to taste

Preparation:

- Pour milk into blender
- Add flax seed
- Add raspberries, cherries & stevia
- Blend until totally smooth

Makes **one** serving

Calories per serving: 121

Pomeberrygranate

Ingredients:

120ml (4 fl.oz) pure pomegranate juice

120ml (4 fl.oz) water

112g (4 oz) frozen mixed berries

Preparation:

- Pour pomegranate juice & water into blender
- Add mixed berries
- Blend until smooth

Makes **one** serving

Calories per serving: 124

Fruity Pea

Ingredients:

56g (2oz) cold cooked peas (from frozen)

120ml (4 fl.oz) pure pineapple juice

168g (6 oz) strawberries

1 medium banana

Ice cubes

Preparation:

- Pour pineapple juice into blender
- Add peas & strawberries
- Chop &add banana
- Add ice cubes
- Blend completely

Makes **two** servings

Calories per serving: 125

Carrot, Mango & Lime Tango

Ingredients:

180ml (6 fl.oz) carrot juice

56g (2 oz) fat-free natural yoghurt

168g (6 oz) frozen mango chunks

1½ tablespoons pure lime juice

2 teaspoons honey

Ice cubes

Preparation:

- Pour carrot juice & yoghurt into blender
- Blend briefly
- Add mango, lime juice & honey
- Pop in ice cubes
- Blend until smooth

Makes **two** servings

Calories per serving: 126

Tomato & Carrot

Ingredients:

240ml (8 fl.oz) tomato juice

2 medium carrots

1 small stick celery

1 tablespoon fresh lemon juice

Pinch of ground black pepper

Pinch of salt

Ice cubes

Preparation:

- Pour tomato juice into blender
- Peel & chop & add carrots
- Blend until smooth
- Chop celery finely & add to mixture
- Add lemon juice, pepper & salt
- Pop in ice cubes
- Blend to combine

Makes **one** serving

Calories per serving: 129

Citrus Smoothie

Ingredients:

180ml (6 fl.oz) pure grapefruit juice

112g (4 oz) fat-free natural yoghurt

1 orange

1tablespoon honey

Preparation:

- Pour grapefruit juice into blender
- Peel & segment the orange & put into blender
- Add yoghurt
- Add honey
- Blend completely

Makes **two** servings

Calories per serving: 129

Gingery Peach

Ingredients:

180ml (6 fl.oz) skimmed milk

60ml (2 fl.oz) water

½ teaspoon ground ginger

168g (6 oz) frozen peach slices

Stevia to taste

Preparation:

- Pour milk & water into blender
- Add ground ginger
- Spoon in peach slices
- Blend until smooth

Makes **one** serving

Calories per serving: 137

Simply Banana

Ingredients:

180ml (6 fl.oz) skimmed milk

1 small ripe banana

½ teaspoon almond extract

½ teaspoon cinnamon

Ice cubes

Preparation:

- Pour skimmed milk into blender
- Chop banana & add to blender
- Add almond extract, cinnamon & ice cubes
- Blend all ingredients

Makes **one** serving

Calories per serving: 140

Blackberry & Cherry Tastebud Tickler

Ingredients:

120ml (4 fl.oz) unsweetened almond milk

84g (3 oz) fat-free natural yoghurt

84g (3 oz) blackberries

84g (3 oz) frozen cherries

½ teaspoon vanilla extract

Preparation:

- Pour almond milk into blender
- Add yoghurt
- Blend briefly to aerate
- Put in raspberries & cherries
- Drop in vanilla extract
- Blend on high setting until completely smooth

Makes **one** serving

Calories per serving: 141

Fruity Veggimix

Ingredients:

240ml (8 fl.oz) pure cranberry juice

112g (4 oz) fat-free natural yoghurt

168g (6 oz) blueberries

84g (3 oz) steamed broccoli (cold)

Ice cubes

Preparation:

- Pour cranberry juice into blender
- Add yoghurt
- Add blueberries & broccoli
- Drop in ice cubes
- Blend until smooth

Makes **two** servings

Calories per serving: 147

Paradise Perfection

Ingredients:

150ml (5 fl.oz) pure orange juice

112g (4 oz) chilled pineapple chunks

56g (2 oz) strawberries

Lots of ice cubes

Preparation:

- Pour orange juice into blender
- Pop in pineapple chunks
- Add strawberries
- Drop in ice cubes
- Blend until smooth

Makes **one** serving

Calories per serving: 149

Ginger Kick

Ingredients:

120ml (4 fl.oz) carrot juice

120ml (4 fl.oz) pure orange juice

1 teaspoon grated ginger root

½ green apple

Ice cubes

Preparation:

- Pour carrot & orange juices into blender
- Add grated ginger root
- Core, chop &add apple
- Drop in ice cubes
- Blend until totally smooth

Makes **one** serving

Calories per serving: 149

Peachy Blackberry

Ingredients:

120ml (4 fl.oz) skimmed milk

2 ripe peaches

84g (3 oz) blackberries

Plenty of ice cubes

Preparation:

- Pour milk into blender
- Remove stones, slice peaches & add to blender
- Add blackberries
- Drop in ice cubes
- Blend everything thoroughly

Makes **one** serving

Calories per serving: 150

Melonectarine

Ingredients:

180ml (6 fl.oz) unsweetened almond milk

1 tablespoon ground flax seed

112g (4 oz) watermelon

1 nectarine

Ice cubes

Preparation:

- Pour milk into blender
- Add flax seed
- Deseed watermelon & add to blender
- De-stone, slice & add nectarine
- Pop in ice cubes
- Blend until totally smooth

Makes **one** serving

Calories per serving: 150

Mangonut

Ingredients:

240ml (8 fl.oz) unsweetened coconut water

168g (6 oz) frozen mango chunks

1 tablespoon pure lime juice

Small pinch cayenne pepper

Ice cubes

Preparation:

- Pour coconut water into blender
- Add mango chunks
- Add lime juice & cayenne pepper
- Put in ice cubes
- Blend to combine

Makes **one** serving

Calories per serving: 154

Orange & Blues

Ingredients:

120ml (4 fl.oz) pure orange juice

112g (4 oz) blueberries

56g (2 oz) fat-free natural yoghurt

½ teaspoon vanilla extract

Ice cubes

Preparation:

- Pour orange juice into blender
- Put in blueberries
- Add yoghurt & vanilla extract
- Blend until everything is combined

Makes **one** serving

Calories per serving: 154

Melemon

Ingredients:

168g (6oz) honeydew melon

56g (2 oz) fat-free natural yoghurt

84g (3 oz) green seedless grapes

½ tablespoon fresh chopped mint

2 teaspoons lemon juice

Ice cubes

Preparation:

- Cut the melon into cubes & place in blender
- Add yoghurt
- Blend the mixture
- Add grapes & mint
- Add ice cubes
- Blend thoroughly

Makes **one** serving

Calories per serving: 155

Melon & Raspberry

Ingredients:

¼ medium cantaloupe melon

56g (2 oz) fat-free natural yoghurt

84g (3 oz) raspberries

Stevia to taste

Ice cubes

Preparation:

- Deseed & cube melon. Put cubes into blender
- Add yoghurt
- Blend briefly
- Add raspberries, stevia & ice cubes
- Blend thoroughly

Makes **one** serving

Calories per serving: 157

Tropical Twister

Ingredients:

180ml (6 fl.oz) pure cranberry juice

1 ripe medium banana

168g (6 oz) frozen mango chunks

112g (4 oz) strawberries

Plenty of ice cubes

Preparation:

- Pour in cranberry juice into blender
- Chop banana & add to blender
- Add mango chunks & strawberries
- Pop in ice cubes
- Blend all ingredients

Makes **two** servings

Calories per serving: 165

Smooth Orange & Cherry

Ingredients:

Juice of 2 oranges

56g (2 oz) fat-free natural yoghurt

112g (4 oz) frozen cherries

1 tablespoon ground flax seed

Plenty of ice cubes

Preparation:

- Pour orange juice into blender
- Add yoghurt
- Drop in ice cubes
- Put in cherries & flax seed
- Blend until smooth

Makes **one** serving

Calories per serving: 165

Banana & Apple Filler

Ingredients:

240ml (8fl.oz) unsweetened almond milk

168g (6 oz) fat-free natural yoghurt

1 ripe medium banana

1 large apple

Preparation:

- Pour almond milk into blender
- Add yoghurt
- Chop & add banana
- Peel, core, slice & add apple
- Blend until smooth

Makes **two** servings

Calories per serving: 166

Fruitful Fantasy

Ingredients:

240ml (8 fl.oz) pure pineapple juice

1 ripe medium banana

112g (4 oz) strawberries

112g (4 oz) chilled pineapple chunks

Pinch of cinnamon

Ice cubes

Preparation:

- Pour pineapple juice into blender
- Chop banana & put into blender
- Add strawberries, pineapple chunks & cinnamon
- Drop in ice cubes
- Blend until smooth

Makes **two** servings

Calories per serving: 166

Spinach Surprise

Ingredients:

336g (12 oz) honeydew melon

28g (1 oz) baby spinach leaves

70g (2 ½ oz) fat-free natural yoghurt

Couple of drops vanilla extract

Ice cubes

Preparation:

- Cut melon into chunks & place in blender
- Add spinach leaves, torn
- Add yoghurt & vanilla extract
- Pop ice cubes in
- Blend until smooth

Makes **one** serving

Calories per serving: 167

Strawberry Surprise

Ingredients:

120ml (4 fl.oz) skimmed milk

112g (4 oz) fat-free natural yoghurt

1teaspoon vanilla extract

168g (6 oz) strawberries

Ice cubes

Preparation:

- Pour milk into blender
- Add yoghurt & vanilla extract
- Pop in strawberries
- Add ice cubes
- Blend until smooth

Makes **one** serving

Calories per serving: 174

Zesty Pinky Lemon

Ingredients:

60ml (2 fl.oz) pure lemon juice

60ml (2 fl.oz) water

84g (3 oz) raspberries

112g (4 oz) fat-free natural yoghurt

1 tablespoon honey

Ice cubes

Preparation:

- Pour lemon juice & water into blender
- Spoon in raspberries
- Blend briefly
- Add yoghurt & honey
- Drop in ice cubes
- Blend until smooth

Makes **one** serving

Calories per serving: 183

Gently Green

Ingredients:

240ml (8 fl.oz) pure apple juice

252g (9 oz) seedless green grapes

56g (2 oz) baby spinach leaves

1 small green apple

Ice cubes

Preparation:

- Pour apple juice into blender
- Pop in grapes
- Add spinach leaves, torn
- Core, chop & add apple
- Add ice cubes
- Blend until smooth

Makes **two** servings

Calories per serving: 184

Veggie Fruity Tooty

Ingredients:

Plenty of ice cubes (or crushed ice)

1 orange

112g (4 oz) peeled cucumber

84g (3 oz) seedless green grapes

56g (2 oz) pineapple pieces

56g (2 oz) chopped carrot

Preparation:

- Put ice into blender & pulse to crush
- Peel, halve, deseed orange & add to ice
- Chop cucumber & add to above
- Add grapes & pineapple
- Blend briefly
- Put in carrot
- Blend everything until completely smooth

Makes **one** serving

Calories per serving: 186

Creamy Tongue-Tickler

Ingredients:

120ml (4 fl.oz) pure orange juice

60ml (2 fl.oz) water

1 small ripe banana

1 teaspoon freshly-grated ginger root

1 teaspoon honey

Ice cubes

Preparation:

- Pour orange juice & water into blender
- Slice & add banana
- Add ginger root
- Spoon in honey
- Add ice cubes
- Blend until smooth & creamy

Makes **one** serving

Calories per serving: 187

Almond Energizer

Ingredients:

240ml (8 fl.oz) unsweetened almond milk

168g (6 oz) fat-free natural yoghurt

168g (6 oz) firm silken tofu

28g (1 oz)) dry roasted almonds

½ teaspoon vanilla extract

Ice cubes

Preparation:

- Pour almond milk into blender
- Add yoghurt, tofu & almonds
- Drop in vanilla extract & ice cubes
- Blend everything until completely smooth

Makes **two** servings

Calories per serving: 196

Spicy Strawberry

Ingredients:

240ml (8 fl.oz) skimmed milk

168g (6 oz) strawberries

1 tablespoon ground flax seed

1 teaspoon cinnamon

1 teaspoon honey

½ teaspoon xanthan gum

Ice cubes

Preparation:

- Pour milk into blender
- Halve & add strawberries
- Add flax seed, cinnamon & honey
- Blend until smooth
- Add xanthan gum & ice cubes
- Blend again

Makes **one** serving

Calories per serving: 210

Summer Refresher

Ingredients:

224g (8 oz) cantaloupe melon

120ml (4 fl.oz) water

1 small banana

1 orange

Ice cubes

Preparation:

- Cube melon & put into blender
- Add water
- Slice & add banana
- Peel, segment & add orange
- Drop in ice cubes
- Blend vigorously

Makes **one** serving

Calories per serving: 212

Orange & Blueberry Buster

Ingredients:

120ml (4 fl.oz) skimmed milk

112g (4 oz) fat-free natural yoghurt

60ml (2 fl.oz) freshly-squeezed orange juice

168g (6 oz)) blueberries

½ teaspoon vanilla extract

Ice cubes

Preparation:

- Pour milk into blender
- Add yoghurt
- Pour in orange juice
- Add blueberries &vanilla extract
- Add ice cubes
- Blend all ingredients thoroughly

Makes **one** serving

Calories per serving: 214

Creamy Dream

Ingredients:

240ml (8 fl.oz) unsweetened almond milk

1 small banana

28g (1 oz) kale leaves (no ribs or stems)

1 tablespoon unsalted peanut butter

½ teaspoon cinnamon

1 teaspoon vanilla extract

½ teaspoon xanthan gum

Preparation:

- Pour almond milk into blender
- Slice & add banana
- Tear & add kale leaves
- Spoon in peanut butter
- Add cinnamon, vanilla & xanthan gum
- Blend until everything is completely smooth

Makes **one** serving

Calories per serving: 216

Pure Pleasure

Ingredients:

120ml (4fl.oz) unsweetened almond milk

112g (4 oz) fat-free natural yoghurt

1 medium banana

84g (3 oz) blackberries

¼ teaspoon vanilla extract

Ice cubes

Preparation:

- Put yoghurt into blender
- Pour in almond milk
- Slice & add banana
- Add blackberries
- Drop in vanilla extract
- Pop in ice cubes
- Blend thoroughly

Makes **one** serving

Calories per serving: 218

Tomato & Mango Tango

Ingredients:

120ml (4 fl.oz) unsweetened almond milk

1 tomato

168g (6 oz) chilled pineapple

168g (6 oz) frozen mango pieces

Ice cubes

Preparation:

- Pour almond milk into blender
- Halve & add tomato
- Chop & add pineapple
- Blend briefly
- Add mango
- Put in ice cubes
- Blend vigorously

Makes **one** serving

Calories per serving: 223

Beety Berries

Ingredients:

60ml (2 fl.oz) freshly squeezed orange juice

56g (2 oz) fat-free Greek yoghurt

56g (2 oz) sliced cooked beetroot

168g (6 oz)) blueberries

84g (3 oz) raspberries

Stevia to taste

Ice cubes

Preparation:

- Pour orange juice into blender
- Add yoghurt
- Blend briefly
- Add beetroot, blueberries & raspberries
- Add stevia & ice cubes
- Blend everything to a smooth consistency

Makes **one** serving

Calories per serving: 231

Green Tea Smoothie Meal

Ingredients:

168g (6 oz) fat-free Greek yoghurt

120ml (4 fl.oz) water

2 teaspoons almond butter

1 teaspoon green leaf tea (or use from green teabag)

½ teaspoon vanilla extract

140g (5 oz) frozen cherries

Preparation:

- Spoon yoghurt into blender
- Add water
- Blend briefly
- Add almond butter
- Put in green tea
- Add vanilla extract & cherries
- Blend until smooth consistency

Makes **one** serving

Calories per serving: 277

Index of Smoothies

Fruit Only

	Calories
Cocomelon	75
Blueberry Sparkle	77
Rhubarb Rocker	94
Passionate Minty Melon	100
Caribbean Calypso	100
Strawberry Delight	111
Berry Mix	117
Pear & Strawberry	118
Berry Nice	120
Pinkalicious	121
Pomeberrygranate	124
Citrus Smoothie	129
Gingery Peach	137
Simply Banana	140
Blackberry & Cherry Tastebud-Tickler	141
Paradise Perfection	149
Ginger Kick	149
Peachy Blackberry	150
Melonectarine	150
Mangonut	154
Orange & Blues	154
Melemon	155
Melon & Raspberry	157
Tropical Twister	165
Smooth Orange & Cherry	165
Banana & Apple Filler	166

Fruitful Fantasy	166
Strawberry Surprise	174
Zesty Pinky Lemon	183
Creamy Tongue-Tickler	187
Almond Energizer	196
Spicy Strawberry	210
Summer Refresher	212
Orange & Blueberry Buster	214
Creamy Dream	216
Pure Pleasure	218
Green Tea Smoothie Meal	277

Fruit & Vegetable

Fruity Watercress	79
Strawberry & Cucumber Cooler	84
Celery & Blueberry	98
Purple Sunset	112
Fruity Pea	125
Carrot, Mango & Lime Tango	126
Fruity Veggimix	147
Spinach Surprise	167
Gently Green	184
Veggie Fruity Tooty	186
Tomato & Mango Tango	223
Beety Berries	231

Vegetable Only

Tomato & Carrot	129

Also by Alicia Brent

A Little Book of Christmas
Resolutions & Reflections for the New Year
Dead Interesting
Samuel Johnson Man of Words
Ellen White Speaks Out